# BOOST YOUR IMMUNE SYSTEM:
# Strengthen your Body and Mind for a Healthy Life

Sylvain MILON

# SUMMARY

# INTRODUCTION

In our modern world, where the challenges of everyday life are many, it is essential to have a strong and resilient immune system. Our immune system is our natural line of defense against disease, infection, and external aggression. Therefore, taking care of our health and strengthening our immunity is crucial to living a fulfilling and healthy life.

This book, "Boost Your Immune System", will guide you step by step to strengthen your body and mind to develop powerful immunity. By understanding how your immune system works, you will be able to take the necessary steps to support and boost it. This book offers practical advice, scientifically proven information and proven techniques to help you reach your full health potential.

The first chapter, "Understanding the Immune System: The Foundation of Health", lays the groundwork by explaining in detail the essential role of the immune system in our body. You will discover how it works, what its different components are, and how it interacts with our environment. By understanding the underlying mechanisms, you will be better equipped to proactively take care of your immune system.

The second chapter, "Healthy Eating for Powerful Immunity: Keys to Enhanced Health," explores the close connection between our diet and our immune system. You will discover the beneficial foods that boost immunity, as well as those that can compromise it. You will be given practical advice on how to eat a balanced and nutritious diet to provide your body with the essential nutrients to support your immune system.

The rest of the chapters will cover other key aspects of boosting your immune system. You'll discover the importance of restful sleep, regular exercise, managing stress and emotions, connecting with nature, and positive thinking. These chapters will provide you with practical tools, expert advice, and inspiring testimonials to help you incorporate these beneficial habits into your daily life.

Join me on this journey to boost your immune system. Together, we will explore ways to strengthen your body and mind, adopt healthy habits and cultivate lasting immunity. Get ready to discover a new perspective on health and embrace the potential of your immune system to live a life full of vitality and well-being.

# CHAPTER 1: "UNDERSTANDING THE IMMUNE SYSTEM: THE FOUNDATION OF HEALTH

Our immune system, the invisible guardian of our body, is more than just a defense mechanism. It is the fundamental pillar of our overall health and well-being. Think of it as a protective shield, constantly on alert to prevent unwanted intrusions and combat threats that could compromise our vital balance.

But what do we really know about this extraordinary system that works tirelessly for our survival? It's time to explore the depths of our immune system and understand its essential role in our lives.

At the heart of our body, the immune system is a complex network of organs, tissues and cells, each playing a crucial role in protecting our health. Our bone marrow produces the stem cells that give rise to our immune soldiers, the white blood cells. These valiant fighters are found throughout our body, ready to intervene as soon as a danger arises.

Among these cells are macrophages, the vigilant guardians that patrol our bodies, engulfing invaders and cleaning up debris. Lymphocytes, on the other hand, are the commanders-in-chief of our immune system, coordinating targeted attacks against pathogens. They fall into two categories: B cells, which are responsible for producing specific antibodies, and T cells, which eliminate infected cells.

But our immune system is not limited to these cells. It also relies on key organs such as the spleen, which filters our blood and detects threats, and the lymph nodes, which serve as communication centers where immune cells exchange vital information. These organs work in perfect symbiosis to ensure the coordination and responsiveness of our immune system.

But it's not just an army of cells in action. Our immune system also has an extraordinary memory. It is able to recognize intruders it has encountered before, allowing it to respond more quickly and effectively to future attacks. This is how vaccines work, by training our immune system to specifically recognize and fight pathogens.

Beyond the science, it is important to understand the emotional aspect of our immune system. Our thoughts, emotions and state of mind can influence how it works. Stress, for example, can weaken our immune system, making it more vulnerable to disease. On the other hand, positive emotions, such as gratitude and joy, can strengthen our immunity and promote optimal health.

To understand our immune system is to understand the magic of our existence. It's about recognizing our body's incredible ability to defend and regenerate itself. It's about realizing that we have the power to actively support our immune system through a healthy, balanced lifestyle.

Throughout this book, we will explore in detail the different facets of our immune system and ways to strengthen it. You'll discover practical tips, stress management techniques, nutritional approaches and much more. Get ready to dive into the depths of your immune system and unleash its extraordinary potential for a lifetime of vibrant health and vitality.

# CHAPTER 2: "HEALTHY FOOD FOR POWERFUL IMMUNITY: THE KEYS TO ENHANCED HEALTH"

Your plate is more than just a food source. It is the fuel that powers your body, providing it with the essential nutrients to support a strong and powerful immune system. Food plays a central role in our health, and understanding the keys to healthy eating is essential to boosting our immunity and living a fulfilling life.

Imagine for a moment that every bite you take is an act of love towards your body. Each carefully selected ingredient is a promise of health and vitality. It's time to explore the beneficial foods that nourish our immune system and discover how to incorporate them into our daily lives in delicious ways.

Colored fruits and vegetables are nutritional gems. Rich in vitamins, minerals and antioxidants, they strengthen our immune system by protecting our cells from free radical damage. Berries, citrus fruits, spinach, peppers and carrots are just a few examples of superfoods that deserve a special place on our plate.

Quality protein is also essential for our immune system. Legumes, nuts, seeds, eggs, fish and lean meats are good sources of protein that provide the amino acids needed to build and repair immune cells. Be sure to include these foods in your meals to optimally support your immune system.

Healthy fats also play a crucial role in a balanced diet. Avocados, walnuts, chia seeds and extra virgin olive oil are rich in beneficial fatty acids, such as omega-3s, that reduce inflammation and boost our immunity. Incorporate them into your dishes and enjoy their benefits for your body and mind.

Also, let's not forget the importance of hydration. Water is the vital element that keeps our immune system in balance. It allows the transport of nutrients, the elimination of toxins and the proper functioning of all body functions. Make sure you drink enough water throughout the day to keep your body hydrated and your immune system in top shape.

Finally, it is important to avoid processed foods that are high in added sugars, saturated fats and artificial additives. These foods can weaken our immune system and compromise our overall health. Choose fresh, unprocessed and organic foods whenever possible to ensure you get the essential nutrients without the harmful substances.

Taking care of our diet is an act of love towards ourselves. Every choice we make has an impact on our health and immune system. Make your plate a source of vitality, pleasure and well-being. Nourish your body with healthy, tasty and nutritious foods, and feel the power of your immunity grow stronger every day.

# CHAPTER 3: "THE IMPORTANCE OF SLEEP TO BOOST YOUR IMMUNE SYSTEM: REGAIN VITAL ENERGY".

Sleep, that enchanted interlude where our bodies rest and regenerate, is much more than a simple break in our hectic lives. It is an essential pillar of our health and well-being, and a powerful ally in strengthening our immune system. When we find restful sleep, we open the doors to vital energy that allows us to face life's challenges with resilience and vitality.

Imagine a night of deep, peaceful sleep, where every cell in your body is bathed in sweet harmony. Your immune system is in action, repairing damage, eliminating toxins and strengthening its defenses. It is during our sleep that our bodies regenerate, our immune systems strengthen and our minds find the rest they need to thrive.

However, in our modern society, sleep is often neglected. We are constantly on the go with screens, work responsibilities and daily concerns. We often sacrifice our sleep time for our commitments, thinking that we can make up for lost sleep later. But in doing so, we deprive our bodies of a vital element for their health and vitality.

Lack of sleep weakens our immune system, making it more vulnerable to infection and disease. It also increases our susceptibility to stress, disrupts our mood and affects our ability to concentrate and make informed decisions. In other words, sleep is the fuel that keeps our bodies and minds functioning optimally.

In order to regain vital energy and strengthen our immune system, sleep is of paramount importance. Here are a few keys to promote quality sleep:

1. Establish a sleep routine: Adopt a regular bedtime and wake-up time, even on weekends. This regularity allows your body to synchronize and optimize the quality of your sleep.

2. Create a sleep-friendly environment: Make sure your room is quiet, dark and well ventilated. Eliminate distractions, such as screens, and create a space where you can relax and rest.

3. Avoid stimulants: Limit your intake of caffeine, alcohol and nicotine, as these substances can disrupt your sleep. Instead, drink soothing herbal teas or warm milk before bed.

4. Establish a relaxing routine: Set up relaxing rituals before bed. This can include reading a book, practicing meditation, breathing exercises or a warm bath. Find what works for you and create a

smooth transition to sleep.

5. Take care of your sleep hygiene: Invest in a comfortable mattress and quality pillows. Create a pre-bedtime hygiene ritual by brushing your teeth, taking a hot shower or practicing gentle stretches.

By paying close attention to our sleep, we open the door to vital energy and enhanced health. Return to the comforting arms of sleep and enjoy the profound benefits it brings to your immune system. Give your body the time it needs to rejuvenate and witness the transformation that occurs when you make sleep a part of your life.

# CHAPTER 4: "PHYSICAL EXERCISE: STRENGTHEN YOUR BODY, STRENGTHEN YOUR IMMUNE SYSTEM"

Exercise, that enchanting dance between our bodies and minds, is more than just a physical activity. It is a powerful way to strengthen our immune system and cultivate optimal health. When we engage in regular practice, we empower our bodies to defend against disease and thrive with vitality.

Imagine yourself in motion, the breath of life flowing through every part of your being. Your body awakens, vibrating with energy and strength. Each movement is a caress to your immune system, giving it the vigor it needs to face the challenges ahead.

Exercise boosts our immune system in several ways. First, it increases blood flow, which allows immune cells to move more efficiently through our bodies to detect and fight infections. In addition, regular exercise reduces stress, which can weaken our immune system. It also improves our overall health, which has a positive impact on our immunity.

There are many forms of physical exercise, and each can provide benefits to our immune system. Cardiovascular training, such as running, swimming or cycling, builds our endurance and stimulates the production of immune cells. Strengthening exercises, such as weight training or yoga, tone our bodies and promote better immune function.

But exercise is not just about physical activity. It is also an opportunity to cultivate a deep connection with our bodies and minds. It is a special time when we can refocus, release stress and nourish our whole being.

By engaging in regular exercise, you give your immune system an emotional boost. You build confidence, self-esteem and mental resilience. Exercise becomes an act of self-love, a way to take care of your body and mind.

Find the activity that resonates with your inner self. Explore different practices and discover what brings you joy and satisfaction. Whether it's dance, yoga, nature hikes or team sports, find your own path to a strengthened immune system.

It is important to note that exercise should be done in a way that is appropriate for your physical condition and abilities. Consult a health care professional or trainer to establish an exercise plan that is right for you and guides you to a safe and beneficial practice.

Take time to move, stretch, sweat and feel the power of your body.

Allow exercise to become an integral part of your life, a source of strength, vitality and support for your immune system.

# CHAPTER 5: "MANAGING STRESS AND EMOTIONS: FREEING YOUR IMMUNE SYSTEM".

Stress, that invisible force that can invade our lives, has a profound impact on our health and immune system. Negative emotions, such as anxiety, anger and sadness, can become a heavy burden to carry, weakening our immune system and making us vulnerable to disease. It's time to free our immune system from the shackles of stress and negative emotions, so we can regain inner balance and flourish.

Imagine for a moment freeing yourself from the weight of stress, worries and negative emotions. You breathe deeply, feeling each breath bring peace and serenity to your body. Your immune system is freed from its chains, ready to defend itself with renewed strength.

Managing stress and emotions is essential to strengthening our immune system. When we are constantly overwhelmed by stress, our bodies produce hormones, such as cortisol, that can weaken our immune system. In addition, negative emotions can disrupt our inner balance and create energy blockages that interfere with the proper functioning of our immune system.

There are many techniques and practices that can help us manage stress and release our emotions, allowing our immune system to thrive. Here are some approaches to consider:

1. Meditation: Meditation is a powerful tool for calming the mind, reducing stress and cultivating conscious presence. Take a few minutes each day to sit in silence, observe your breathing and let your thoughts dissipate. Regular meditation can help strengthen your immune system and promote a state of inner balance.

2. Conscious breathing: Become aware of your breathing and practice deep, slow breathing techniques to relax. Conscious breathing helps regulate the nervous system, reducing stress and strengthening our immune system.

3. Emotional expression: Find healthy ways to express your emotions, whether through writing, dancing, painting or speaking. Release what is buried inside of you, allowing your immune system to break free from the grip of negative emotions.

4. Yoga practice: Yoga is a combination of physical exercise, breathing and meditation that promotes better stress management and mind-body harmony. Practice yoga regularly to strengthen your immune system and create inner balance.

5. Regular physical activity: Exercise is a great way to release stress and stimulate the production of endorphins, the feel-good hormones. Find a physical activity you enjoy and make it part of

your daily routine.

6. Social connection: Cultivate healthy, positive relationships with others. Social support and empathetic listening can help reduce stress and strengthen our immune system.

Take time to reconnect with yourself, listen to yourself and take care of your emotional needs. Free your immune system from the shackles of stress and negative emotions, and allow your body to thrive in a state of calm and balance. You deserve a life where joy, peace and health merge in perfect harmony.

# CHAPTER 6: "THE BENEFITS OF NATURE: IMMUNITY NURTURED BY THE ENVIRONMENT

Nature, this majestic cradle of life, is much more than just a setting. It is an infinite reservoir of benefits for our health and immune system. When we connect with nature, we nourish our whole being, harmonize our energy and strengthen our immunity.

Imagine yourself surrounded by the lush beauty of nature. You breathe in the fresh air, smelling the delicate scent of wild flowers. The sun's rays caress your skin, bringing you warmth and vitality. You feel in harmony with the world around you, your immune system awakening with each moment of communion with nature.

Nature offers a multitude of benefits for our immune system. First of all, it is an inexhaustible source of vitamins, minerals and antioxidants essential to our health. By eating fresh, organic foods from the earth, we strengthen our immune system from the inside out.

In addition to diet, simply spending time in nature can have a positive impact on our immune system. The practice of "forest bathing," also known as shinrin-yoku, is an ancient Japanese method of taking a slow, mindful walk in the woods. This practice reduces stress, lowers blood pressure and increases the production of immune cells.

Nature also offers us the opportunity to engage in physical activities outdoors. Whether it's hiking, biking, swimming or gardening, these activities allow us to connect with our bodies, strengthen our immune system and release endorphins, the happy hormones.

But nature is more than just a tool to strengthen our immune system. It is a source of wonder, calm and comfort to our emotional being. When we immerse ourselves in the natural beauty that surrounds us, we let our worries fade away and find a refuge in the present moment. This reduces stress, frees our immune system from emotional strain and allows us to return to a state of inner balance.

It is important to find moments to connect with nature in our daily lives. Even short moments spent observing the flowers in a garden, feeling the grass under our bare feet, or contemplating a sunset can have a profound impact on our well-being and immunity.

Take time to reconnect with nature. Take regular trips to parks, forests or the water's edge. Care for the plants and animals that share our world. Allow your immune system to thrive in the nourishing energy of nature.

Remember, we are intrinsically connected to nature. By reconnecting with it, we find our true essence and strengthen our immune system in a holistic way. Embrace the magic of nature and let it guide your path to flourishing health and inner harmony.

# CHAPTER 7: "THE POWER OF POSITIVE THINKING: CULTIVATE A HEALTHY MIND FOR FORTIFIED IMMUNITY"

Positive thinking, that bright inner force that can transform our perception of the world, is a powerful ally in strengthening our immune system. By cultivating a healthy, optimistic mindset, we create an environment conducive to healing, resilience and vitality. It's time to explore the power of positive thinking and pave the way to fortified immunity.

Imagine yourself enveloped by the softness of positive thoughts that light up your mind. You feel a warmth that penetrates you, nourishing every cell in your body. Your immune system awakens to this new perspective, vibrating with energy and vitality.

Positive thinking has a profound impact on our immune system. When we cultivate optimistic and caring thoughts, our bodies respond by producing endorphins, hormones that promote well-being and strengthen our immune system. In addition, positive thinking reduces stress, which can weaken our immunity, and promotes a state of inner balance that is conducive to health.

But positive thinking is not limited to a simple affirmation of oneself or a forced smile. It is a true state of mind, a way of seeing and understanding the world around us. It involves cultivating an attitude of openness, gratitude and compassion towards oneself and others.

Here are some strategies for cultivating positive thinking and strengthening your immune system:

1. Practice gratitude: Take time each day to write down the things you are grateful for. It can be simple moments of joy, positive relationships, or even lessons learned from difficult times. Gratitude feeds our spirit and strengthens our immune system.

2. Eliminate negativity: Pay attention to negative thoughts and limiting thought patterns. Identify them and replace them with positive affirmations. Cultivate a caring and supportive inner dialogue that supports your emotional well-being and builds immunity.

3. Surround yourself with positivity: Choose to spend time with positive and inspiring people. Read books, listen to podcasts or watch videos that lift your spirit and encourage you to see the best in yourself and the world.

4. Practice self-compassion: Be gentle with yourself and treat yourself with kindness. Accept your imperfections and mistakes, and remind yourself that you deserve love and respect. Self-compassion feeds your spirit and strengthens your immune system.

5. Visualize healing: Practice creative visualization by imagining your immune system vibrating with health and vitality. Visualize yourself in perfect health, full of energy and vitality. This practice strengthens your spirit and creates an alignment between your mind and body.

Positive thinking is a powerful key to strengthening your immune system. By cultivating a healthy, optimistic and caring mindset, you create an environment conducive to healing, resilience and vitality. Allow positive thinking to guide your path to strengthened immunity and a fulfilling life.

Chapter 8: "Daily Habits for Sustainable Health: A Boosted Immune System Forever"

We've come to the final chapter of this journey to a stronger immune system. Through the various steps we've explored, you've discovered valuable knowledge and practices that can transform your health and well-being. Now, it's time to build on these insights and adopt daily habits to maintain a boosted immune system forever.

The habits we cultivate every day are the foundation of our long-term health. It is these small, repeated actions that, accumulated over time, have a huge impact on our immune system. So, what are those daily rituals that will keep your immune system strong and resilient?

1. Balanced diet: Continue to focus on a healthy, balanced diet. Eat a variety of fresh fruits and vegetables, lean proteins, whole grains and healthy fats. Be sure to include foods rich in essential nutrients such as vitamins C, D and E, zinc and antioxidants. Make

every meal an opportunity to nourish your body and support your immunity.

2. Regular physical activity: Maintain a regular exercise routine. Whether it's walking, running, yoga, dancing or any other activity you enjoy, the important thing is to move your body every day. Regular exercise boosts your immune system, reduces stress and gives you vital energy.

3. Restorative sleep: Put a premium on the quality of your sleep. Make sure you get a good night's sleep by creating a soothing bedtime routine, avoiding screens before bed and promoting a restful environment. Sleep is an essential part of regenerating your immune system and maintaining optimal health.

4. Stress management: Continue to cultivate stress management practices that help you find inner balance. Whether it's meditation, deep breathing, journaling or other relaxation techniques, take time each day to connect with yourself and release built-up tension. Managing stress is an important key to maintaining a strong immune system.

5. Social Connection: Remember the importance of social relationships in your life. Cultivate positive and nurturing connections with your family, friends and community. Share moments of joy, exchange and mutual support. Social connection helps strengthen your immune system by providing a sense of belonging and emotional well-being.

6. Overall health: Continue to take care of your overall health. Avoid smoking, limit alcohol consumption and avoid toxic substances. Be sure to maintain good personal hygiene, stay well hydrated and take care of your environment to create a healthy

space that supports your well-being.

By adopting these daily habits, you will create a lifestyle that nourishes and strengthens your immune system. Every little bit helps, and together they build a protective shield for your long-term health.

I encourage you to put these teachings into practice in your daily life. Incorporate them into your routine with love and kindness for yourself. You have the power to cultivate lasting health and a boosted immune system forever.

Continue to embrace the path to health and embody the infinite potential of your immune system. You are an extraordinary being, full of strength and resilience. Nourish yourself with these daily habits and shine your inner light, for you deserve a life of health and happiness.

# CONCLUSION
## A Healthy Life: Strengthen your Body and Mind

Congratulations! You have taken an extraordinary journey through the pages of this book, exploring the different dimensions of health and discovering concrete ways to strengthen your body and mind for a lifetime of good health. You've taken the time to immerse yourself in knowledge, explore new practices and integrate positive habits into your daily life. You are now ready to fully embrace your potential and live a life of radiant health and well-being.

On this journey, you have come to understand that health is not just the absence of disease, but a harmonious balance between your body, your mind and your environment. You have learned that your immune system is a precious treasure, an inner force that protects, heals and nourishes your entire being.

You've discovered that healthy eating, regular physical activity, restful sleep, stress management, connecting with nature, positive thinking and daily habits are the fundamental pillars for strengthening your immune system and living a fulfilling life.

But remember, dear reader, this book is more than just a guide. It is a call to action, an invitation to transform your life. Health is an ongoing journey, a constant dance between yourself and your well-being. There may be ups and downs, challenges and moments of doubt, but always remember your inner power.

You have the power to create a healthy life. You are the hero of your own story. Every choice you make, every thought you cultivate, every action you take is a step closer to thriving health.

Never forget that you deserve a vibrant life filled with vitality, joy and fulfillment. Take care of yourself, listen to your body, nourish your spirit and honor your unique self.

I wish you all the best on your journey to a healthy life. May each day be a new opportunity to rise, grow and shine. You have all the tools you need to succeed. So move forward with confidence, passion and love.

Strengthen your body and mind, embrace the beauty of health and live a fulfilling life. You are ready to conquer the world with your life energy. Embrace this new adventure and spread your light wherever you go.

Happy trails to a healthy life!